6 Ingredient Recipes for NO-MEAT Athletes

Vegan, Whole Food, High Protein, Low Cost, Easy!

Andrew Blakehall
(Vegan Athlete)

Published by Iditatran Press (USA) 948 Hudson Street, New York, NY 10014,
(Australia) Iditatran Press 19489 Wollumburah St. Sydney NSW,
Australia, (Canada) edition Iditatran, 2010, 39 Rue De Filbraet,
Montreal, Quebec, Canada, M4P 24, (England) 39 Brighton, F2CR OLA

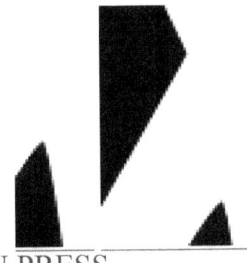

IDITATRAN PRESS

Tempeh Stir Fry
No Moussaka Wraps
Collard Wraps
Garbanzo Magic
Hobo Beans and Salsa
Wild Rice and Beans with Broccoli
Quinoa & Vegetables
Rosemary Garlic Sweet Potatoes
Quick Salad
Fake Meat warps
Vegan Nacho's
In a Rush Shake
Veggie Sausage with Brussels
Sprout's
Simple Oatmeal
Brown Rice and Split Pea Gruel
Epic Beet and Split Pea Soup
Natto and Rice
Healthy Ice Cream
Almond Apple Chips
Simple Stir Fry

Tempeh Stir Fry
Cooking time: 11 minutes

Ingredients:
1 package tempeh
6-8 stalks kale, chopped or 1 cup spinach, chopped
2 garlic cloves, minced
½ onion, sliced thin
½ red bell pepper
1 Lemon

Directions:
1. In medium saucepan, heat 1 Tsp. of Olive oil on medium-high heat.
2. Add garlic and onion. Add a dash of water as needed to prevent burning.
2. After about 2 minutes, add red bell pepper and stir. You may need to add a dash of water.
3. After about 1 minute, add tempeh.
4. After about 3 minutes, add kale and cover for about 5 minutes.
5. Garnish with lemon squeeze, sriracha, and Braggs amino acid.

No Moussaka Wraps
Cooking time: 18 minutes

Ingredients:
1½ can white beans, strained
8 kale or collard leaves
1 eggplant, sliced into 1/8 inch chips
1 zucchini, sliced into 1/8 inch chips
1 red bell pepper, sliced thin
¼ onion, sliced thin
1 lemon (not required but recommended)

Directions:
1. Preheat oven to 400 degrees.
2. Lightly grease baking tray with olive oil.
3. Place vegetables in tray, let cook for about 13 minutes,
4. Stir vegetables, add beans, place in oven for 5 minutes.
5. Remove from oven, place all ingredients in food processor and blend with juice of lemon or dash of water.
Place on collard leaf, add Tabasco and nutritional yeast to taste.

Collard Wraps
Cook time: 5 minutes

Ingredients:
6 Large Collard green leaves
3 Large carrots, blanched
1 avocado
1 cucumber, skinned and sliced thin
½ red bell pepper, cut thin
½ lemon

Directions:
1. Start by mashing the avocado into a paste with 1 Tbsn. of water.
2. Lay the collard leaves flat and apply a small spoonful of avocado to the center.
3. Layer carrots, cucumber, and bell pepper. Squeeze lemon over the top. Roll together.
4. Add Braggs Amino's to taste.

Garbanzo Magic

Cooking time: 4 minutes.

Ingredients:

1 -1½ can(s) garbanzo beans, strained and washed
1 can corn niblets, strained and washed
1 small avocado, diced
1 cup spinach, washed

Directions:

1. Place garbanzo beans and corn in pan, heat until warm.
2. Place in bowl with spinach and avocado.
3. Stir bowl.
4. Add sriracha, Tabasco, or Balsalmic vinegar to taste.

Hobo Beans and Salsa
Cook time: 3 minutes

Ingredients:
1- 1½ can(s) black beans, strained and washed
¼ small onion, diced
1 Roma tomato, diced
1 small avocado, diced

Directions:
1. Place black beans in pan, heat until warm.
2. Place in bowl with other ingredients.
3. Add Sriracha, Tabasco or juice of Lime to taste

Wild Rice and Beans with Broccoli

Cook time: 4 minutes or 18 minutes, (depending on if you're using leftover rice or you're making rice fresh)

Ingredients:

1 cup of wild rice, (purchase in bulk food section)
1 can kidney beans, strained and washed
1 cup broccoli, chopped into florets
1 clove garlic, minced thin

Directions:

1. Cook rice in pot.
2. Warm up beans in saucepan or microwave.
3. In Pot #2 Steam broccoli and garlic. (Note broccoli takes about 90 seconds to cook, so if you're making the rice fresh, wait until it's finished before you start the broccoli.)
4. Combine ingredients and add Bragg's Aminos and/or Sriracha and/or Nutritional Yeast.

Quinoa & Vegetables
Cook time: about 10 minutes

Ingredients:
1 cup quinoa
10 Brussels sprouts, sliced *or* 1 cup broccoli, sliced
½ red bell pepper, sliced thin
1 carrot, *shaved (Julienned thin)*
1 avocado, sliced
1 lemon

Directions:
1. Prepare quinoa in pot #1. It should take about 7 minutes from the time you place it in boiling water. Make sure you cover the pot with lid.
2. In pot #2 steam Brussels sprouts (5 minutes) or broccoli (about ninety seconds) Make sure you cover either selection with a lid.
3. Strain both pots.
4. Add all ingredients and flavor with juice of lemon and Bragg's Aminos or Sriracha.

Rosemary Garlic Sweet Potatoes

Cook Time: 40 minutes.
Despite the long cook time, the prep is actually very easy.

Ingredients:

2 large sweet potatoes (or Yams) cut into 1/8' wedges
3 garlic cloves, diced
1 can black beans, washed and strained
2 sprigs fresh rosemary, chopped fine
1 Tsp. coconut oil or olive oil (this ingredient cannot be substituted, so if you are looking for a zero oil recipe, this one won't work.)

Directions:

1. Preheat oven to 450 degrees.
2. Grease baking pan with olive oil.
3. Place sweet potatoes on baking sheet and place in oven.
4. Wait about 15 minutes.
5. After approximately 15 minutes, bring 1 tablespoon of coconut oil to medium heat in frying pan.
6. Place garlic in frying pan.
7. Wait about twenty seconds, add dash of water (this cools the pan and prevents the garlic from burning.)
8. Add rosemary, 'swirl' saucepan (or stir with ladle) so contents brown on all sides.

9. When garlic is brown (should take about 1 minute of cooking) remove sweet potatoes from oven and drizzle with garlic\rosemary\olive oil. Use a spoon to distribute evenly.

10. Place Sweet Potatoes back in oven. It should take *about* another 15-25 minutes to cook, but I recommend checking every ten minutes to make sure. Sweet potatoes are done when you can easily stick a spoon into the meat and see steam rise.

11 Heat beans in pan (no oil required.) When they are ready (about 90 seconds) remove Sweet Potatoes from oven and distribute beans on top.

Tip: Often the thin pieces will cook more quickly than the thick pieces, so sometimes I will take out all thin pieces and eat them while the thick slices cook for a few more minutes.

Tip: I recommend mustard and ketchup on these babies.

Quick Salad
Cook time: 5 minutes

Ingredients:
1 cup spinach, washed
1 tomato, diced
1 cup firm tofu, cubed (optional)
1 apple, sliced or ¼ cup sunflower seeds or ¼ cup raisins
1 tspn. Balsalmic vinegar
1 Lemon

Directions:
1. Heat saucepan on high heat (no oil necessary).
2. Add tofu, while it is cooking, toss all ingredients together.
3. When tofu is browning, squeeze lemon on top.
4. Place Tofu in with salad and toss.

Fake Meat warps.*
Prep time: 15 seconds.

Ingredients:
1 box of your favorite vegan deli slices (I recommend tofurkey)
1 small avocado
Optional but recommended:
1 package single serving Seaweed sheets (available at Trader Joe's for 99c)
2 packs mustard

Directions:
1. Squeeze mustard onto deli slice.
2. Squeeze avocado onto deli slice.
3. Add 1 Sheet of Seaweed
4. Roll.

*This is one of my only recipes that is not a whole food, however, I felt I had to include it. It's high in protein, inexpensive, fast, and tastes amazing. If you're ever near a Trader Joes, give it a try.

Vegan Nacho's
Cooking and prep time 14 minutes.

Ingredients:
¼ bag tortilla chips
1 package vegan cheese
1 can black beans, strained or 1 can refried beans
½ onion, diced
1 avocado, cubed
1 tomato, diced or ¼ cup chopped cilantro

Directions:
1. Preheat oven to 350 degrees.
2. Heat 1 Tspn. Olive oil on medium-high heat.
3. Add onions, cook for about two minutes, adding dashes of water and stirring as necessary.
4. Add beans (if you use refried beans you'll want to add 1 Tbsn. of water and stir)
5. While beans are cooking, place chips on tray.
6. Distribute beans and cheese over chips.
7. Place tray in oven for about 10 minutes (You will want to check every five minutes to prevent burning.)
8. When it's finished, garnish with tomato and avocado.
Add Tabasco or Sriracha to taste.

In a Rush Shake

Ingredients:
2 scoops vegan protein powder
1 banana
1½ cup non-dairy milk or water
1 tspn flax seed oil (optional)
2 ice cubes (optional)
1 dash cinnamon (optional)

Directions:
Combine all ingredients and blend.
Pour and enjoy!
(Don't forget to soak the blender jug before
your run out the door!)

Veggie Sausage with Brussels Sprouts

Cook time: 11 minutes

Ingredients:

2 veggie sausage links (I recommend Tofurkey)
15 Brussels sprouts, diced
3 cloves garlic, minced
¼ white onion, chopped thin

Directions:

In a large saucepan, heat 1 tspn. of either coconut oil or olive oil.
2. Add garlic and a dash a water.
3. After about 1 minute, add onions and a dash of water.
4. Stir.
5. Add Brussels sprouts and ¼ cup of water, stir and cover.
6. After about four minutes, add sausage, immediately reduce heat to low, stir and cover.
7. After about six minutes, serve and enjoy.
8. Garnish with ketchup and Nutritional Yeast or with Bragg's Amino Acids and Sriracha.

Simple Oatmeal
Cooking time: 8 minutes

Ingredients:
½ cup oats
1 banana, diced
½ cup almond milk
¼ cup raisins
Dash cinnamon
1 scoop Vanilla flavored Vegan Protein
supplement (optional)

Directions:
1. Boil 2 cups of water on high.
2. Add oats.
3. Immediately reduce heat to medium low.
4. Add Raisins and cinnamon.
5. Add Banana***
6. Cover pot.
7. Wait about eight minutes, stirring
occasionally.
8. Pour into bowl and add Almond Milk.
9. If you add protein powder do it at the
very end.

*** I like adding my banana about halfway
through the cooking process, this gets it
soft and mushy. Some people prefer to add
it at the very end with the almond milk,
either is fine.

Brown Rice and Split Pea Gruel

Cooking time: 21 minutes if you're making from scratch, 3 minutes if you have rice and split peas pre-cooked.

Ingredients:

1 cup brown rice
1 cup split peas
Dash cayenne pepper or black pepper
Dash olive oil
Dash Nutritional Yeast

Directions:

1. Prepare brown rice and split peas in separate pots.
2. When they are ready, strain 90% of the water.
3. Add to blender with other ingredients, blend on high.

Epic Beet and Split Pea Soup
Prep time: 35 minutes

Ingredients:
This one takes a bit longer to prepare, but it's well worth it.
2 large beets, quartered
1 cup split peas
1 cup non-sweetened almond milk
4 carrots, diced
½ white onion diced
2 cloves garlic, minced
1 tspn. coconut oil (you can substitute water, but I don't recommend it)

Directions:
1. In Pot #1: boil all vegetables together *except* garlic and onion
2. In Pot #2: boil split peas.
3. In saucepan: Heat 1 Tsp. coconut oil, add garlic and onion and sauté on high heat for about 2 minutes, add water to the pan, reduce heat to medium and stir until onion is brown. When it is ready, set aside.
4. When Pot #1 and #2 are finished, strain 90% of the water.
5. Pour 1 cup Almond milk into blender with contents of all pots.
6. Blend on high.

Natto and Rice
Cook time: 12 minutes.

Hailing from Japan, Natto is a food staple that all vegans should be familiar with. It is high in protein and may be the highest available source of vitamin B-12 found in non-meat products. It can be found in most Japanese markets, or many world supermarkets, such as Uwajamia. Many people hate it the first time they eat it. But if you stick with it, it will grow on you!

Ingredients:
1 package natto
1 cup white rice
1 dash of Nori flakes or soy sauce.

Directions:
1. Prepare rice.
2. Add Natto.
3. Season with Nori or Bragg's Amino Acids.

Healthy Ice cream
Prep time: 5 minutes (if you have bananas ready)

Ingredients:
7 slightly browning bananas, peeled
3-5 strawberries,
1 Cup plain almond milk
Dash cinnamon
Vegan protein powder (optional)

Directions:
1. Peel bananas and place in plastic bag.
2. Place in freezer and leave to freeze for at least six hours.
3. Place frozen contents in blender with plain almond milk.
4. Blend.
5. Gradually add or reduce almond milk to achieve desired thickness.
6. Add cinnamon.
Serve and enjoy

High Fat, Almond Apple Chips
Prep time: 90 seconds

Ingredients:
2 green or red apples or pears washed and
sliced into 'chips'
¼ cup non-sweetened Almond butter
(Do not substitute peanut butter)

Directions:
Smear apple slices with a thin sheen of almond
butter.

Simple Stir Fry
Cook time: 10 minutes

Ingredients:
1 cup firm tofu or Seitein
1 Cup Brussels sprouts, sliced thin
4 Asparagus spears, sliced
½ Red bell pepper, sliced
3 Garlic cloves, minced
Orange (optional)

Directions:
1. Heat 1 Tsp. olive oil or coconut oil on medium high heat in saucepan or wok.
2. Add garlic.
3. Add dash of water and stir for 1 minute.
4. Add Seiten and stir for 4 minutes (you may need to add a little water)
5. Add bell pepper and stir for 2 minutes.
6. Add asparagus and stir for 2 minutes.
7. Reduce heat to low, stir, and cover for five minutes.
8. Add Braggs Amino's to taste.
9. If you have an orange lying around, feel free to squeeze it over the dish, the juice gives a nice sweetness.